I0413035

Paleo Diet Cookbook

All you ever need to know about Paleo Diet

AMARPREET SINGH

Publisher - The Thought Flame

THE THOUGHT FLAME

TURNING SPARK INTO FLAME

info@thethoughtflame.com

www.thethoughtflame.com

Table of Contents

Introduction

Have you wondered how many people are able to live healthier and much longer lives just by switching over to the Paleo Diet? What is so special about this diet anyway? How does it work so well with your body to show these kinds of results?

The answers to these questions are very simple? The only reason why the Paleo diet works alongside your body's normal function rather than against them and that can help you lose weight over time is because you are working with your body's most natural instinct. You see, thousands of years ago our ancestors ate a special way: hunting the animals around them, cooking their meals and stuffing themselves with the variety of vegetation nearby. The Paleo Diet works the same way, utilizing healthy and lean meat, fruits, vegetables and nuts to help your body get back to those ancestral routes.

In this eBook you will learn exactly how the Paleo Diet can help you not only keep your weight to a healthy and reasonable level, but how it can help you fight off and prevent a wide range of common diseases. You will also find 25 of the most delicious Paleo Diet recipes you will ever come across and that will certainly help to kick off your new diet on a good note.

I invite you to come and explore the many benefits that the Paleo Diet has to offer you and your family. Without further ado, let's hop into Chapter One.

Chapter One: What Is The Paleo Diet?

The Paleo Diet is considered to be one of the healthiest diet that you can follow today and it is one that many people who are trying to achieve a healthier lifestyle follow on a daily basis. The Paleo Diet is the only diet that works by following your natural genetic instincts in such a way that it will help you to stay in shape and energetic. Unlike the Paleo diet, many of the foods that we consume today contain unhealthy trans fats and sugars, which has been found to cause many diseases in the human body such as diabetes, cancer, obesity and heart disease.

There are many foods that you can have while on the Paleo Diet while other foods you need to avoid entirely. Some of the foods that you can have while following this diet include:

- Seafood

- Plenty of Lean Meats

- Healthy Sources of Fat

- Vegetables

- Fruits

- Nuts

- Seeds

Some of the foods that you should avoid at all cost while on the Paleo Diet include:

- Grains

- Alcohol

- Legumes

- Dairy

- Sugar

- Processed Foods

- Starches

How To Build The Perfect Paleo Diet

There are many healthy foods that you can consume while following the Paleo Diet and many of the foods that you can have can easily be used to create the most delicious recipes for.

1. Lean Proteins-whenever you add lean proteins to your diet as they help to enhance the strength of your bones and increase your immune system function. Aside from those benefits, lean protein sources can also help you feel full longer in between meals.

2. Vegetables and Fruits-we all know that fruits and vegetables are especially healthy for us. Both fruits and vegetables are packed with healthy antioxidants and contain important minerals and vitamins. These substances help your body to fight off and prevent common diseases that can occur in people such as diabetes and cancer.

3. Healthy Fat Sources-yes, there is such a thing known as a healthy fat source. The main source of healthy fats that you should try to aim for to include in your diet is known as an Omega 3 fatty acid. And Monounsaturated Fats This acid has been known to help reduce the chance of diabetes, heart disease, cancer and even obesity.

The Benefits of The Paleo Diet

It is no secret that the Paleo Diet helps you to get the weight loss results that you are looking for. Not only will the Paleo Diet help you to lose weight in the long run, but it will also help you to improve your overall blood health and to improve your entire immune system.

The one downside to the Paleo Diet is that many people are willing to follow the recommendations of a diet from other people. Naturally, people are hesitant to try something new. Many people need to know exactly why a diet works and how it works before they begin trying it out for themselves. This is understandable and I am here to tell you everything that you need to know about the Paleo Diet.

There are many health benefits of following the Paleo Diet and that include:

- Increase your daily intake of important vitamins and minerals.

- Increase the amount of antioxidants that you take in.

- Have an increase in energy.

- Feel better physically, emotionally and mentally in the long run.

The Truth About The Paleo Diet

There is a common misconception about the Paleo Diet such as that it doesn't really even work. I am here to tell you that is absolutely false. Since this diet is rarely heard of and talked about, there are many questions that are bound to pop up. Here are some common questions that have been asked about this diet and here are some of the most truthful answers that you will find.

1. Does This Diet Actually Work To Help Manage and prevent Diabetes?

The answer to this question is that yes, the Paleo Diet can help you to manage your diabetes or prevent diabetes altogether. In fact, there have been numerous studies conducted on the diet itself to see how it worked for people suffering from diabetes. In this study it was found that a majority of the people used for the test were able to reverse their diabetic signs and symptoms of Type 2 Diabetes. Some were able to recovered from the disease altogether and never suffered from diabetes after that.

2. Does the Paleo Diet Help To Alleviate Cardio Vascular Disease?

According to the Center For Disease Control, cardiovascular disease is the number one cause of death in the United States today and that number of people who die every year from these diseases continues to grow. Scientists found that when our ancestors ate the same kind of foods that are included in the Paleo diet, virtually none of them suffered from either a heart attack or stroke. The reason behind these amazing results comes down to one thing: back then our ancestors did not put anything greasy or fatty into their diet in order to make their food taste good. Our ancestors kept their diet as simple as possible and that is exactly what the Paleo Diet does today.

3. How Does The Paleo Diet Help With Autoimmunity?

The term autoimmunity refers to the circumstance where the body's own immune system begins to attack the body itself. This is a disease where the immune system is not acting as it should. Normally our immune systems are supposed to protect us from foreign invaders such as a number of viruses, bacterial infections and parasites. In this case the immune system will view the entire body as a threat and try its best to get rid of it.

The perfect example of this is during an organ transplant. During this kind of procedure the number one concern is that the body will reject the organ. Because of this concern a patient will start to undergo many medications meant to lower their auto immune response to give the organ a surviving chance within the body.

There are multiple instances where autoimmunity begins to get out of control and can lead to several common diseases such as Multiple Sclerosis, Lupus and Rheumatoid Arthritis. By sticking to a healthy Paleo Diet and specifically sticking to the Autoimmune protocol of the diet, you can help boost your autoimmune response and to help it recognize the parts of your own body that are not a threat. This can help you fight off other autoimmune responses in the long run.

Chapter Two: A Few Slow Cooker Tips

One of the most useful and helpful tools that you can have in your kitchen today is a slow cooker. A slow cooker cannot only save you lots of time, but it is also a helpful tool that is extremely easy to use. Anybody can use a slow cooker, whether you are an advanced chef or just a beginner. Literally all that you have to do in order to use it is to fill it up and turn it on. That is it.

If you have never used a slow cooker before, here are some helpful tips that every slow cooker owner needs to know.

Helpful Tips

1. You will have only two primary settings on your slow cooker to help cook your food: Low

and High. The temperature will range for these two settings as Low will be about 200 degrees Fahrenheit and the high setting will be about 300 degrees Fahrenheit.

2. Cooking your food one hour on the highest setting equals to about 2 to 2 ½ hours on the lowest setting.

3. Whenever you cook your food in your slow cooker, whatever you do, DO NOT REMOVE THE LID! If you do, you will lose about 15 to 20 minutes in cooking time as your slow cooker will need to regain the steam and heat it has lost when the lid was removed.

4. For recipes that call for you to brown the meat and sauté vegetables before you add them into your slow cooker will help you to enhance the overall flavor of your entire dish. While most people choose to skip this step, it helps to improve the taste of your meal in the long run.

5. When using seasoning in your food keep these important details in mind:

- Using whole or whole leaf herbs will improve in flavor as you cook your meal.

- Using ground seasoning in your food will only cause your food to lose flavor as it cooks.

- It is best to only add ground seasoning right after your meal has finished cooking to help improve the flavor of the dish in the long run.

6. To make great tasting side dishes, you should always utilize the slow cooker.

7. If you have made a dish that is much soupier than you would like it to be, all that you have to do is place your dial on high once you have finished cooking so the excess liquid can evaporate.

8. It is best to use the cheapest and less tender meats that you can in your slow cooker. When you cook meat in a slow cooker for 6 to 8 hours, it ends up becoming much more tender than you ever could have hoped.

9. During the summer months it is best to cook primarily with your slow cooker. Not only will it help you to keep your house cool during these crucial months, but it will also help you to save money on your gas bill for a couple of months.

10. You can easily purchase low cost slow cooker lines to help you with easy clean up after you use your slow cooker. If you do not want to purchase liners, cooking spray will work just as good.

11. Keep in mind that food that is left cooking on the bottom of your slow cooker pan will cook much faster than the rest of the dish. The bottom of your pan is the perfect place to cook your meat and vegetables to give them more

flavor and tenderness in the long run.

12. If you are using vegetables it is best to make sure they are all cut at the same length and width. This will help cook them much more evenly.

13. If you are using tender vegetables in your dish such as Zucchini, Tomatoes and Mushrooms, it is best to add them to your dish during the last hour of cooking.

14. If you fill your Crockpot to the brim with food, the entire dish will not cook properly. It is best to only fill your Crockpot up either ½ or ¾ of the way to allow your food adequate time to cook better. If you only fill your slow cooker up less than ½ way full, your food could possibly burn as it will cook much faster.

15. Always try to find a slow cooker that is best for you. There are so many different brands and kinds of slow cookers out there, your

choice are limitless. Before you purchase on doing your research first before finding the perfect one for you.

Now that you know some helpful tips that will help you make the most out of your slow cooker, it is time to start making some delicious Paleo Diet slow cooker recipes!

Delicious Paleo Diet Slowcooker Recipes

Savory Chicken Musakhan

If you love the cuisine from Palestine, you are going to love this dish. This dish comes from the heart of Palestine tradition and will introduce new flavors that you will instantly fall in love this. Using a Paleo Diet. This classic dish combines savory ingredients such as chicken, pine nuts and delicious saffron, making this dish a potential family favorite.

Serving Size: 6

Preparation Time: 6 hours and 10 minutes

Ingredients:

-2 Pounds of Boneless and Skinless Chicken Thighs

-¼ tsp. of Cloves, Ground

-¼ tsp. Allspice, Ground

-1.5 Tbsp. of Olive Oil

-A handful of Pine Nuts

-Pepper and Salt For Taste

-2 Whole Onions, Sliced Thinly

-1 tsp. of Cinnamon, Ground

-Pinch of Saffron

-Fresh Ming Leaves, To be Used As Garnish

Directions:

1. In a microwave safe bowl combine your onions, cinnamon, olive oil, ground cloves and saffron. Toss until thoroughly combined. Place this bowl into your microwave and heat up for 2 minutes, 30 seconds. Stir and microwave again at 2 minutes, 30 seconds.

2. Place your chicken thighs into your slowcooker and season lightly with some salt and pepper for taste. Next add in your microwave onion mixture and stir thoroughly until evenly mixed.

3. Place on the lowest setting and cover. Cook for the next 6 hours or until chicken is tender.

4. Next sauté your pine nuts in a little bit of olive oil until they are browned. Add some salt and pepper for taste and sprinkle over some chicken.

5. Serve your chicken and top with fresh mint and pine nuts. Enjoy.

Melt In Your Mouth Pork Spare Ribs

This recipe makes perfect spare ribs that taste better than they smell. The great tasting ribs that are popular in Asian culture inspired this recipe and these ribs will come out practically falling off of the bone. You can easily serve these with a side of steamed white rice or serve these as a complete side dish.

Serving Size: 4

Preparation Time: 6 hours and 10 minutes

Ingredients:

-2 to 4 cups of Vinegar, White

-4 pounds of Pork Ribs

-1 tsp. of Pure Sea Salt

-1 tsp. of Garlic Powder

-Dash of Salt and Pepper For Taste

-2 Cups of Water

-Dash of Asian Seasoning For Taste

-2 Tbsp. of Apple Cider Vinegar

-3 Tbsp. of Coconut Aminos

Directions:

1. Pour your white wine and water over your spare rib. Sprinkle with a dash of sea salt and mix thoroughly until fully combined. Let your spare ribs soak overnight or for the next 12 hours.

2. Once the soaking period is over, drain your ribs completely. Then seasoning your spare ribs with some more sea salt, pepper and a dash of garlic powder. Next make sure to coat both sides of your ribs thoroughly with some Asian seasoning.

3. Place your spare ribs upright in your slowcooker. Then add your apple cider vinegar and coconut aminos to the bottom of your slowcooker. Cover with lid.

4. Cook on the highest setting for the next 4 to 6 hours or until most of the liquid has

evaporated from the slowcooker.

5. Serve as a main dish or serve with a bowl of steaming rice and enjoy.

Savory Slowcooker Pot Roast

No slowcooker cookbook is complete without its own unique pot roast recipe. The reason why pot roasts are so popular is simply because you are able to combine all of your important meal bases in one simple dish. This recipe comes out absolutely amazing and includes all of your favorite ingredients such as cauliflower and potatoes. Feel free to add your own ingredients and to be as creative as you wish.

Serving Size: 6

Preparation Time: 8 Hours and 40 minutes

Ingredients:

-4 Pounds of Beef, Chuck Roast

-1 Tbsp. of Olive Oil

-4 Garlic Cloves, Diced and Crushed

-1 cup of Wine, Red

-10 Sprigs of Thyme, Fresh

-1 Carrot, Peeled and Sliced Into Small Chunks

-2 Celery Stalks, Sliced Into Small Chunks

-1 Bay Leaf

-1 Small Onion, Sliced Into Thin Pieces

-1 Small Cauliflower, Leaves Removed First and Cut Into Tiny Pieces

-Dash of Salt and Pepper For Taste

Directions:

1. Season your beef chuck roast with some salt and pepper. In a separate saucepan add some

olive oil and heat over high heat. Swirl the olive oil to evenly coat the pan and add your beef to it. Heat the beef until it develops a nice brown crust on all sides. Continue until completely seared. Then add your beef to your slowcooker.

2. Next pour in your red wine into your still hot saucepan and add to slowcooker over your beef.

3. Next add your fresh thyme, garlic and bay leaf to your slowcooker and stir until thoroughly combined. Add in the remaining ingredients except for the cauliflower. Season your mixture with a dash of pepper and salt.

4. Cook on the highest setting for the next 4 to 6 hours. Once you have 1 hour remaining in the cooking process add in your cauliflower and finish cooking.

5. Serve while still piping hot and enjoy.

Traditional Puerco Pibil

This is a delicious traditional Mexican dish made with a little Paleo style thrown into it. While this dish uses pork shoulder, which is very meat-centric, there are not many vegetables used. Feel free to serve this dish up with a side of steamed vegetables or a healthy soup. This dish is great to make when you are having a busy day and just want to come home to a home cooked meal.

Serving Size: 4

Preparation Time: 8 hours and 10 minutes

Ingredients:

-1 Whole Onion, Sliced Thinly

-1 tsp. of Black Pepper, Ground

-1 tsp. of Salt

-1, 15 Ounce Can of Tomatoes, Diced and Fire Roasted

-1 tsp. of Cumin, Ground

-2 Tbsp. of Paprika

-2 tsp. of Salt

-1 Whole Orange, Juiced

-5 Pounds of Pork Shoulder

-¼ Cup of Apple Cider Vinegar

-Dash of Nutmeg

Directions:

1. In a small mixing bowl mix your paprika, cumin, 1 tsp. of Salt, dash of nutmeg and black pepper. Stir until thoroughly combine and add a touch of water to blend well until the seasonings form a paste.

2. Next slice your onion into thin slices and sauté in a separate saucepan with some olive oil

until onions are translucent. Next add in your can of tomatoes and cook with onions until tomatoes are soft.

3. Trim the fat off of your pork shoulder and slice the pork into thin slices. Season the pork with a dash of salt and pepper.

4. In your slowcooker pour in your orange juice and apple cider vinegar and stir until thoroughly combined. Next add in your seasoning paste and stir in your slowcooker until it fully dissolves. Add your pork into the slowcooker next and top with your onion and tomato mixture.

5. Cover with a lid and cook on the lowest setting for the next 6 to 8 hours.

6. Serve for breakfast, lunch or dinner and thoroughly enjoy.

Slowcooker Style Honey Garlic Chicken Wings

If you are a fan of chicken wings, you are going to love these honey garlic chicken wing recipe. While you are following a very healthy diet, you don't have to worry about not eating delicious meals. This is a simple recipe to follow and perfect to make during your favorite football game or family party.

Serving Size: 3

Preparation Time: 6 hours and 10 minutes

Ingredients:

-3 Pounds of Boneless Chicken Wings (Feel free to use more if your slowcooker can hold more)

-½ tsp. of Sea Salt

-½ tsp. of Pepper, Ground

-¾ Cup of Honey, Liquid

-2 Tbsp. of Olive Oil

-1 ½ Tbsp. of Garlic, Minced

Directions:

1. Place your boneless chicken wings into a slowcooker.

2. In a separate mixing bowl mix your honey, garlic, salt, ground pepper and olive oil until all the ingredients are well blended.

3. Drizzle your honey mixture over your wings until the sauce covers your wings entirely.

4. Cook your wings on the lowest setting for the next 6 hours or 3-4 hours on the highest setting.

Hawaiian Style Pulled Pork

This recipe is perfect for those who do not like to spend too much time preparing their meals as this dish only uses 3 simple ingredients. Remember, whatever dishes you decide to make that will follow the Paleo diet, it is better to keep it as simple as possible. With this dish it is as simple as it gets and it tastes great too.

Serving Size: 6

Preparation Time: 6 hours and 5 minutes

Ingredients:

-4 Pounds of Fresh Pork Shoulder

-2 Tbsp. of Fresh Ginger

-1 Can of Pineapple, Cubed or Crushed

Directions:

1. Place your fresh pork shoulder into your Crockpot

2. Add your entire can of pineapple into your slowcooker, juices and all. Next add in your ginger. Stir until thoroughly combined

3. Cover and cook on the lowest setting for the next 6 to 8 hours.

Savory Balsamic Chicken and Spicy Sausages

With this dish you will not only have a meal that tastes great, but that is great to look at on your plate. While it is unheard of to combine two meats together in a Paleo Diet recipe, this will give you the chance to have something savory and spicy at the same time while still eating healthy. Feel free to add your own favorite ingredients to spice up this dish some more.

Serving Size: 6

Preparation Time: 5 to 7 hours and 10 minutes

Ingredients:

-4 Chicken Breasts, Skinless and Boneless

-1 Whole White Onion, Sliced Thinly

-6 Cloves of Garlic, Chopped

-6 Italian Sausage Links (Feel free to use spicy links or sweet links)

-Dab of Virgin Olive Oil

-1 tsp. of Salt

-1 tsp. of Italian Seasoning

-1 tsp. of Garlic Powder

-½ Cup of Vinegar, Balsamic

-1 tsp. of Additional Italian Seasoning

-1 Cup of Chicken Stock

-2, 14. 5 Ounce Cans of Organic Tomatoes, Diced

-1, 15 Ounce Can of Tomato Sauce

-½ tsp. of Additional Salt

-½ tsp. of Additional Garlic Powder

Directions:

1. Lay your chicken breasts at the bottom of your slowcooker and drizzle a touch of Olive Oil on top of it. Next add in your 1 tsp. of Garlic Powder, Italian Seasoning and Salt without mixing it to combine. Just sprinkle it on top of your chicken.

2. On top of your chicken add your sausage links. On top of your sausages add in your onion and freshly chopped garlic. On top of that add in your diced tomatoes, chicken stock, vinegar and tomato sauce. Last add in other seasonings. Again, do not mix.

3. Cover your slowcooker and cook on the highest setting for the next 5 hours or on the lowest setting for the next 7 hours. Serve while piping hot and enjoy thoroughly.

Apple Spiced Pork Tenderloin

Pork tenderloin is probably the most affordable and savory kind of meat that you can ever buy. Adding apples to your pork in this recipe gives it a sweet, yet savory flavor, which is sure to please even the pickiest of eaters. This is a great dish to make whenever you want to impress your guests and is a great meal to make whenever you are having a busy day.

Serving Size: 4

Preparation Time: 8 hours and 15 minutes

Ingredients:

-Dash of Nutmeg

-2 Pounds of Pork Tenderloin

-2 Tbsp. of Honey, Raw

-4 Fresh Gala Apples

Directions:

1. Prepare your Gala Apples by slicing and coring them. Place your apple slices into the bottom of your slowcooker and sprinkle them with a dash of nutmeg.

2. Prepare your pork tenderloin by slicing it in half and placing it on top of your apple within your slowcooker. If you have any remaining apple slices, place these on top of your pork tenderloin and sprinkle with some additional nutmeg.

3. Cover and cook on the lowest setting for the next 8 hours. Serve as soon as it is finished cooking.

Slowcooker Style Carnitas

It is no secret that pork comes out tasting amazing whenever you make it in a slowcooker.

In this dish you will utilize limes and oranges, which give these carnitas a special kick. This dish is perfect to make whenever you are craving Mexican food and are a great way to stay healthy. You can add your favorite toppings or ingredients if you wish.

Serving Size: 5

Preparation Time: 5 hours and 15 minutes

Ingredients:

-4 to 5 Pounds of Roast Pork Loin

-2 Whole Oranges

-1 Whole Lime

-1 tsp. of Garlic Powder

-1 tsp. of Chili Powder

-1 tsp. of Salt

-1 tsp. of Cumin, Ground

-1 Tbsp. of Adobo

-2 Cups of Organic Chicken Stock

-4 Cloves of Garlic, Crushed

-1 Source of Healthy Fat of Your Choice

Directions:

1. Slice your pork roast into 2" slice. Make sure to trim the fat prior to cooking.

2. Mix your garlic powder, salt, adobo and chili powder together until thoroughly combined. Toss this seasoning over your pork steaks.

3. In a separate saucepan add the healthy fat of your choice and heat it up. Sear your pork steaks until browned. Once pork is browned move to your slowcooker.

4. After your pork is seared combine your chicken stock, crushed garlic and tomato paste. Add to your saucepan and het thoroughly. Once heated add to your slowcooker, making sure to

scrape the pan as you go.

5. Next juice both your lime and oranges and drizzle over your pork.

6. Cover your slowcooker and cook on the lowest setting for the next 5 hours. Enjoy.

Italian Style Beef Sandwiches

If you miss the taste of bread ever since you started the Paleo diet, now you can get something that is as close to the real thing. With this recipe you will be able to have a great tasting "sandwich" without the bread. This is a Paleo diet friendly recipe that looks and tastes great.

Serving Size: 2

Preparation Time: 7 to 8 hours and 20 minutes

Ingredients:

-2 Pounds of Beef Chuck Roast

-1 tsp. of Oregano, Dried

-1 tsp. of Basil, Dried

-½ tsp. of Salt

-1 tsp. of Rosemary, Crushed and Dried

-1 tsp. of Onion Powder

-1 tsp. of Garlic Powder

-½ Cup of Water

-¼ tsp. of Pepper, Ground

-6 Large Portobello Mushrooms, Just the Caps

-2 Tbsp. of Dijon Mustard

Directions:

1. Heat a touch of olive oil in a saucepan over medium heat while you combine your oregano, basil, salt, garlic powder, onion powder,

rosemary and pepper together. Sprinkle over your roast.

2. In your heated saucepan sear your roast on all sides until thoroughly browed.

3. Place into your slowcooker with water and cover. Cook on the lowest setting for the next 7 to 8 hours.

4. Once fully cooked take out your roast and shred into small pieces using two forks. Dump remaining water and add your Dijon mustard. Place shredded beef back into slowcooker and stir with mustard until thoroughly combined. Heat for an additional 10 minutes. Place your mushroom caps into your saucepan with some olive oil, salt and pepper and roast for 15 minutes.

5. Using the mushroom caps as your "buns" place shredded beef between them. Enjoy.

Delicious Slowcooker Style Cinnamon Chicken

If you are looking for the perfect savory dish to satisfy your taste buds, you are going to love this cinnamon chicken made slowcooker style. Combining the perfect blend of cinnamon and other spices, this chicken comes out both sweet and spicy. This dish is perfect to make when you don't have the time to make a traditional meal or when you just want to make something easy.

Serving Size: 4

Preparation Time: 6 hours and 5 minutes

Ingredients:

-2 Pounds of Chicken Breasts, Boneless Is Ideal

-2 tsp. of Paprika

-2 Whole Bell Peppers of Your Choice, Thinly

Sliced

-2 tsp. of Cinnamon

-1 Whole Onion, Diced Into Small Pieces

-¼ tsp. of Nutmeg

-1 Cup of Organic Chicken Broth

-4 Cloves of Garlic, Minced

Directions:

1. Combine all of your ingredients into a Ziploc freezer bag, including the chicken. Seal, making sure all of the air is out and place into your freezer for the night. The next day defrost your meal.

2. Pour all of the contents into your slowcooker and cook on the lowest setting for the next 6 hours. You can also cook this dish on the highest setting for 4 hours.

3. Serve with a salad and enjoy.

Greek Style Stuffed Chicken Breasts

This is the perfect dish to make especially for lovers of Greek cuisine. A great recipe to make if you want to impress your friends or if you simply want to spoil yourself. While this dish uses feta feel free to leave it out if you are not a fan. Great to serve with a side of steamed vegetables or a fresh helping of salad.

Serving Size: 4 to 6

Preparation Time: 6 to 8 hours and 20 minutes

Ingredients:

-4 to 6 Chicken Breasts, Boneless

-1 Tbsp. of Healthy Oil of Your Choice

-½ of Red Pepper, Sliced Thinly

-½ of an Onion, Diced

-6 Ounces of Fresh Spinach Leaves

-2 Pepperoncini Peppers, Sliced Thinly

-1 ½ tsp. of Oregano, Fresh

-Dash of Salt and Pepper For Taste

-Squeeze of a Lemon

-2 tsp. of Garlic, Minced

-1 Cup of Organic Chicken Stock

-1/3 Cup of Feta Cheese (optional)

-½ cup of Wine, White

-1 tsp. of Parsley, Fresh

Directions:

1. Cut a deep hole at the end of each chicken breast to form a deep pocket then season both sides of the chicken with some salt and pepper. Set aside.

2. In a separate saucepan pour a dab of olive oil and sauté your peppers and onions until the onions are translucent. Next add in your fresh spinach leaves and garlic and cook long enough for the spinach to wilt. Next add in your oregano and some salt and pepper. Mix thoroughly until thoroughly combined.

3. If you are using feta cheese stuff a good amount into the inside of your chicken pocket of each breast. Then spoon in your spinach mixture into the pockets of your chicken breast. Sprinkle some fresh lemon juice over the top of your chicken and place chicken into your slowcooker. Add in your chicken stock and wine.

4. Cover your slowcooker and cook on the lowest setting for the next 6 to 8 hours. Serve and enjoy.

Tasty Cranapple Turkey Breast

Who says that you have to have turkey only on Thanksgiving? Not only will you be able to enjoy turkey whenever you want, but the cranberries and apples that you will use will give this dish a sweet tasting flavor. This recipe is perfect if served alongside a side of steaming veggies and will surely impress your entire family

Serving Size: 6

Preparation Time: 6 to 8 hours and 5 minutes

Ingredients:

-½ Cup of Maple Syrup

-6 Pound Turkey Breast, Bone-In

-Dash of Salt for Taste

-3 Whole Apples, Peeled, Cored and Sliced Thinly

-½ Cup of Vinegar, Apple Cider

-4 Cups of Cranberries, Rinsed

Directions:

1. Place your entire turkey breast into your slowcooker and season generously with some salt.

2. Next surround your turkey with your sliced apples and cranberries. Then pour your apple cider vinegar and syrup over the top of your turkey breast.

3. Cover your slowcooker and cook on the lowest setting for the next 6 to 8 hours or until the fruits are softened and the meat is cooked completely. Serve with veggies and enjoy.

Caramelized Plantains with Shredded Pork

If you are looking for the easiest shredded pork recipe, this is the recipe for you. With this recipe you won't need to add any side dishes as the plantains compliment the pork nicely. You can even make this dish more delicious by adding a few slices of fresh avocado on top. Not only is this dish healthy, but it tastes amazing.

Serving Size: 6

Preparation Time: 8 to 10 hours and 45 minutes

Ingredients For Your Pork:

-2 Pounds of Pork Loin

-3 Cups of Beef Broth

-1 tsp. of Onion Powder

-Dash of Salt and Pepper For Taste

-1 Yellow Onion, Diced Into Small Pieces

-1 Tbsp. of Garlic Powder

Ingredients For Your Plantains:

-4 Brown Colored Plantains, Peeled and Sliced lengthwise

-1 tsp. of Cinnamon

-Dash of Salt

-Dash of Allspice

-2 Tbsp. of Fresh Coconut Oil

-4 Tbsp. of Coconut Milk, Canned

Directions:

1. Add all of the ingredients needed for your pork into your slowcooker and for on the lowest setting for the next 8 to 10 hours. As soon as the pork is down, shred your pork using two forks.

2. In a separate saucepan add your coconut oil and heat up. Once heated add in your plantains. Sprinkle the top of those plantains with your salt, cinnamon and allspice. Cook the plantains for the next 4-5 minutes per side until they become soft.

3. Next add your cooked plantains to a food processor and puree until it is smooth.

4. Serve your plantains and shredded pork together and garnish with fresh avocado slices and enjoy.

Spicy Jambalaya Soup

If you are needing to bring some spice into your life, this is the perfect way to do it. This soup is not only healthy, but it brings together a great mix of seasoning that is delicious. Feel free to change up the ingredients as you wish or to substitute ingredients for other. This is the perfect dish to make on a rainy afternoon or whenever you want to make something that is easy.

Serving Size: 4

Preparation Time: 6 hours and 50 minutes

Ingredients:

-5 Cups of Organic Chicken Stock

-2 Bay Leaves

-1 Onion, Chopped

-2 Cloves of Garlic, Diced and Crushed

-4 Ounces of Chicken, Boneless and Diced

-4 Peppers of Your Choice, Chopped Finely

-1 Pound of Shrimp, De-veined

-1 Head of Cauliflower

-3 Tbsp. of Cajun Seasoning

-¼ of Hot Sauce of Your Choice

-2 Ounces of Sausages, Diced

Directions:

1. Place your peppers, garlic, chicken, hot sauce, onions, Cajun seasoning, organic chicken stock and bay leaves into your slowcooker. Cover and cook on the lowest setting for the next 6 hours.

2. When you have 30 minutes left in the cooking process add in your diced sausages. Cover.

3. Dice up your cauliflower until it resembles rice and when there is 20 minutes left in the cooking process add this into your slowcooker.

4. Once the soup has finished cooking, spoon into bowls and enjoy.

Savory Braised Chilean Beef

This recipe allows you to be as versatile as you want. You can easily use this dish to serve as a whole roast or can use it to make something as simple as tacos. Made using the right combination of spices, you will easily fall in love with this dish. Since this recipe is very versatile you can allow yourself to let your inner chef out and to become as creative as you want. Add in whatever additional ingredients you like to make this dish even more delicious.

Serving Size: 6

Preparation Time: 8 hours and 5 minutes

Ingredients:

-1 Whole Beef Roast.

-2 tsp. of Cocoa Powder

-1/8 tsp. of Cinnamon

-1 tsp. of Cumin

-4 Cloves of Garlic, Minced

-1 tsp. of Oregano

-3 Tbsp. of Chili Powder

-1 Tbsp. of Vinegar, Balsamic

-Half of a Red Onion, Cut Into Thick Slices

-Dash of Salt and Pepper For Taste

-½ tsp. of Chipotle Powder

-¾ Cup of Freshly Brewed Coffer

Directions:

1. Combine all of your ingredients except for your coffee vinegar, beef and onion until thoroughly combined. Add enough water into your ingredients until you are able to form a thin paste. Using this paste rub onto your beef on all sides.

2. On the bottom of your slowcooker add a thin layer of your onions and place your beef roast on top of it. Stir your coffee and vinegar together until thoroughly combined and pour over your beef roast.

3. Cook on the lowest setting for the next 6 to 8 hours or until the meat is nice and tender. Serve with a side of steamed vegetables and thoroughly enjoy.

Succulent Lamb Roast

Most people who follow the Paleo Diet have yet to incorporate lamb into any of their meals. If you are not used to eating lamb, it is something that can be a little off-putting at first, but once you have it enough you will begin to crave it. This recipe helps to make your transition to a lamb dish much easier and will leave you wanting more. Add with your choice of a side or a salad.

Serving Size: 4

Preparation Time: 7 hours and 10 minutes

Ingredients:

-2 Pounds of Fresh Lamb Roast

-1 Tbsp. of Cumin, Ground

-1 Tbsp. of Paprika

-1, 14.5 Ounce Can of Tomatoes, Diced and Fire Roasted

-1 tsp. of Garlic Powder

-1 tsp. of Chili Powder

-1 Pack of Diced Bell Peppers, Frozen

-Salt and Pepper For Taste

Directions:

1. Place your whole lamb roast into your slowcooker. Next pour in your peppers and tomatoes around the lamb roast.

2. Next add in your paprika, chili powder, salt, pepper, garlic powder and cumin to your slowcooker. Stir until your lamb roast and tomatoes are evenly coated. Cover.

3. Cook your meal on the lowest setting for the next 7 hours.

4. Once the meat is fully cooked, take your lamb out and shred apart using two forks and serve.

Slowcooker Style Kimchi Chicken

If you have not heard of Kimchi or have never tried it, you will fall in love with this recipe. Kimchi is one of the most valued foods in Korea and is used in many main dishes and side dishes in the country. With this dish you will be able to give your chicken intense and delicious taste when using the kimchi. Not only will it give your chicken a good and spicy kick, but it will leave your family wanting more of it.

Serving Size: 4

Preparation Time: 6 hours and 25 minutes

Ingredients:

-1 Cup of Organic Chicken Broth

-2 Pounds of Chicken Thighs, Boneless and Skinless

-2 Cups of Cabbage Kimchi, Drained

-4 Scallions, Sliced Into Small Slices

-1 Tbsp. of Sesame Oil, Dark

-6 Garlic Cloves, Minced

-1 tsp. of Ginger, Minced or Grated

-1 Tbsp. of Soy Sauce

-2 tsp. of Sugar Sweetener of Your Choice

Directions:

1. Mix all of your ingredients except for your scallions, kimchi and chicken and place into your slowcooker.

2. Place your chicken thighs into your slowcooker and nestle it into the center. Spoon your sauce mixture over the top of it.

3. Cover your slowcooker and cook for the next 4 to 6 hours on the lowest setting.

4. Once your meal has finished cooking, set your slowcooker to the highest setting then add your kimchi. Cook for an additional 20 minutes and serve. Top with scallions and enjoy.

Traditional Beef Tongue in Roasted Pepper Sauce

I know that beef tongue is probably something you have never tried, but now that you are on the Paleo Diet it is time to broaden your horizons. Organ meats are especially nutritious for you as they are packed with lots of protein and if it is prepared correctly, you won't be able to tell the different between that and beef chunks. Following the Paleo diet means going back to our ancestral routes and nothing does it better than this recipe.

Serving Size: 4

Preparation Time: 8 hours and 10 minutes

Ingredients For The Beef Tongue:

-1 Beef Tongue

-3 Bay Leaves

-Dash of Sea Salt and Pepper For Taste

-1 Large Onion, Thinly Sliced

-3 Cloves of Garlic, Crushed or Minced

-Water, Enough of It So It Covers The Entire Tongue

Ingredients For The Sauce:

-1 Red Pepper, Roasted, Diced and Peeled

-1 Large Onion, Diced

-1 tsp. of Thyme

-1 tsp. of Oregano

-Dash of Salt and Pepper For Taste

-3 Cloves of Garlic, Minced

-20 Ounces of Tomatoes, Sliced Into Small Pieces

-1 Serrano Chili Pepper, Roasted and Diced

-6 Ounces of Tomato Paste

Directions For Beef Tongue:

1. Wash the beef tongue thoroughly under running cold water. Pat dry.

2. On the bottom of your slowcooker line it with a layer of your sliced onions, crushed or minced garlic and bay leaves.

3. On top of that layer add your beef tongue and season it with a dash of salt and pepper.

4. Submerge your beef tongue in enough water and cover your slowcooker.

5. Cook the beef tongue for the next 8 hours on the lowest setting and remove from your slowcooker. Remove the skin of the beef tongue as well upon completion.

6. Using two forks shred the beef tongue and mix with prepared sauce.

Directions For Sauce:

1. In a separate saucepan, heat your pan with some healthy oil over medium heat. Add in your onions, red pepper, Serrano chili and garlic. Sauté until onions turn translucent.

2. Add in what remaining ingredients you have into the saucepan and stir until thoroughly combined.

3. Reduce your heat and allow sauce to simmer for 30 minutes.

4. Once finished pour sauce over shredded beef tongue and enjoy.

Traditional Style Meatballs and Spaghetti

When on the Paleo Diet it is important for you to learn how to adapt your favorite foods into foods that are Paleo friendly. This is just one of those recipes. While both spaghetti and bread are not Paleo friendly and many traditional spaghetti dishes require you to use one of the two in some form or another, we have a recipe that you will love to make on a daily basis. In this recipe you will use grain-free meatballs and wheat-free spaghetti, allowing for a nutritious and filling meal without breaking your diet. With the added benefit of using your slowcooker, you won't have to worry about dealing with a mound of dishes once you have finished cooking.

Serving Size: 4

Preparation Time: 5 hours and 5 minutes

Ingredients:

-1 Spaghetti Squash, Medium In Size

-1 Pound of Italian Sausage, Ground

-6 Cloves of Garlic, Left Whole

-2 tsp. of Italian Seasoning

-1, 14 Ounce Can of Tomato Sauce

-2 Tbsp. of Relish, Hot Pepper

-2 Tbsp. of Olive Oil

Directions:

1. Place your tomato sauce, hot pepper relish, garlic, Italian Seasoning and olive into your slowcooker and stir until thoroughly combined.

2. Next place you will need to cut your squash in half and scoop out all of the seeds. Once

done place both pieces of your squash into your slowcooker.

3. Next roll your meat into small meatballs and fit as many as your slowcooker can fit inside around your squash.

4. Cover and cook on the lowest setting for 5 hours.

5. Take your squash out and using a fork, pull lengthwise to make "spaghetti." Top this "spaghetti you're your meatballs and your sauce. Garnish with a touch of parsley and serve.

Classic Slowcooker Chicken Mirepoix

This dish is a great way to get a traditional French meal without having to pay a ton of money for it. If you have never heard of the term Mirepoix, it is just a fancy way of saying the dish contains carrots, celery and onion. This is the perfect dish to have when you need to feel full as it is stuffed with equal amount of vegetables and meat. You can impress your friends with this dish or make it when you want to have a romantic dinner with your spouse.

Serving Size: 4

Preparation Time: 6 hours and 5 minutes

Ingredients:

-1 Chicken, Whole

-2 Large Carrots, Peeled and Diced Into Small Pieces

-Dash of Sea Salt

-3 Cloves of Garlic, Crushed

-Dash of Black Pepper, Ground

-2 Large Stalks of Celery, Diced Into Small

Pieces

-Juice of 1 Lemon

-1 Onion, Chopped Finely

-5 Small Sprigs of Thyme, Fresh and 3 Sprigs Diced Into Fine Pieces

Directions:

1. Wash your whole chicken under running cold water and pat dry with a napkin.

2. Season your chicken generously with some salt and pepper, both on the inside and the outside.

3. In your slowcooker cover the bottom with a layer of only half of the vegetables that you have diced. Then lay your whole chicken on top of it.

4. Next place half of your crushed garlic with 2 whole sprigs of thyme inside of the chicken. Then sprinkle the remaining thyme and

crushed garlic over the top of the chicken.

5. Pour a little fresh lemon juice over your chicken. Cut lemon into slices and place into inside of chicken. Cover your slowcooker.

6. Cook on the lowest setting for the next 6 hours, slice up chicken and serve with cooked vegetables. Enjoy.

Classic Cabbage and Corned Beef

The best part about owning a slowcooker and following the Paleo Diet is that you never have to worry about missing out on the holidays. While this is a traditional Irish meal and is usually served on St. Patty's Day, you can enjoy this dish whenever you wish. Not only is this dish packed with healthy protein and vegetable sources, it tastes just like it would in Ireland. Make this to impress your friend's on St. Patty's day or make as a Sunday night dinner with a fresh cup of ale.

Serving Size: 4

Preparation Time: 8 to 9 hours and 5 minutes

Ingredients:

-2 to 3 Cups of Water

-1 Cabbage, Cut Into Wedges

-6 Large Carrots, Peeled and Sliced Into Thick Chunks

-3 Pounds of Fresh Corned Beef Brisket

-1 Packet of Corned Beef Seasoning Mix

-2 Large Onions, Peeled and Chopped Finely

Directions:

1. In your slowcooker add in your chopped cabbage, carrots and onion. Stir together until thoroughly combined.

2. Rinse your corned beef under running cold water and then pat dry with a paper towel. Next add it into your slowcooker on top of vegetable. Season the corned beef with seasoning mix.

3. Pour your water over the corned beef and cover your slowcooker.

4. Cook on the lowest setting for the next 8 to 9 hours or until brisket is tender. Serve while still piping hot and enjoy.

Sweet Barbeque and Honey Spare Ribs

It does not matter what you do to them, pork spare ribs taste delicious regardless. With this recipe you will be able to make the most succulent and sweet spare ribs you have ever tasted. Perfectly served with a side of asparagus, your taste buds and your stomach will be satisfied. If you are looking to serve the most delicious ribs on Football Sunday or when you are just craving good home cooked BBQ, this is the recipe for you.

Serving Size: 3

Preparation Time: 8 hours and 10 minutes

Ingredients For Barbeque Sauce:

-4 Cloves of Garlic, Minced

-Healthy Cooking Oil of Your Choice

-1 tsp. of Sea Salt

-1 tsp. of Cumin, Ground

-1 tsp. of Basil, Dried

-1 tsp. of Mustard, Dry

-½ tsp. of Cayenne Pepper

-1 cup of Onion, Minced

-1 tsp. of Oregano, Dried

-2 Tbsp. of Vinegar, Apple Cider

-2 Tbsp. of Honey

-1 Cup of Tomato Paste

-1 ½ Cup of Organic Chicken Broth

Ingredients For Spare Ribs:

-Dash of Salt and Pepper For Taste

-4 Pounds of Pork Spare Ribs

Directions:

1. In a separate saucepan, heat up some oil and sauté your onions until they turn translucent. Next add in all of your herbs and spices and stir until thoroughly combined and smooth in texture. Bring your onion mixture to a low boil and remove from heat.

2. Season your spare ribs with a dash of salt and pepper for taste and place into your slowcooker so that they are laying evenly.

3. Pour your onion sauce as evenly as you can

over your ribs and cover.

4. Cook on the lowest setting for 8 hours or until the meat is practically falling off of the bone.

5. Serve with some roasted asparagus as a side and thoroughly enjoy.

Fresh Cucumber Noodles Topped With Strawberry Vinaigrette

This is one of the best and great tasting appetizer that you can make and that will surely please all of your guests. With limited ingredients you won't need to slave over this recipe for hours on end. Even the Strawberry Vinaigrette is extremely easy to make. As a healthy appetizer, this recipe will help you and your guest to feel slightly full so you won't have to worry about over-eating at dinner. Easy to make and simply delicious.

Serving Size: 2

Preparation Time: 30 minutes

Ingredients:

-1 Cucumber

-2 Tbsp. of Vinegar, balsamic

-1 Tbsp. of Dijon Mustard

-8 Large Strawberries, Cut Into Quarters and With Tops Removed

-Small Pinch of Sea Salt and Black Pepper For Taste

-1 Lemon, Used For Garnish

-1 1/3 Tbsp. of Olive Oil, Extra Virgin

Directions:

1. Using a sharp knife cut your cucumber lengthwise and cut into thinly sliced "noodles." Set aside.

2. Using a food processor puree your olive oil, strawberries, salt, pepper, balsamic vinegar and mustard until it is a smooth consistency. Place in your slowcooker. Cover

3. Cook your Puree sauce for 15 to 20 minutes or until warm.

4. Place your newly made cucumber noodles into a bowl and spoon warm puree mixture on top. Toss to coat evenly. Make sure to enjoy.

Savory Coconut and Pumpkin Roasted Soup

During the fall everybody is crazy over the taste of pumpkin. Pumpkin is a great ingredient to use in practically anything that you can make from salads, entrees to soups. This is one recipe that actually calls for you to use real pumpkin and is still one of the easiest dishes that you can make. So, make sure you grab extra pumpkins when looking for your jack-o-lantern because you won't be able to get enough of this recipe.

Serving Size: 2

Preparation Time: 6 hours and 30 minutes

Ingredients:

-1 Small Pumpkin, 4 Total Cups of Pumpkin Flesh

-1 Tbsp. of Butter

-4 Cups of Organic Chicken Stock

-2 tsp. of Cumin

-1 tsp. of Ginger, Ground

-½ tsp. of Red Pepper Flakes

-2 Medium Sized Carrots, Peeled and Chopped Into Small Pieces

-1 Small Pear, Peeled, Cored and Chopped Into

Small Pieces

-1 Small Can of Coconut Milk

Directions:

1. Add 4 cups of Mashed Pumpkin (once you have cut your pumpkin into small pieces) and place into your slowcooker. Next add in the rest of your ingredients and cover your slowcooker.

2. Cook on the lowest setting for the next 5 to 6 hours. Once fully cooked add your soup to a food processor to puree it and achieve the consistency that you want.

3. Garnish with a few pumpkin seeds if you want and enjoy.

<u>Conclusion</u>

Hopefully you have found some of the best Paleo friendly recipes that you will ever lay your eyes on. There are plenty of Paleo style breakfast, lunch, dinner and dessert recipes here that you can make to impress your friends or family.

I know that being on a Paleo diet can seem like a torture spell and a punishment for you, but that could not be any further from the truth. As long as you try your best to spice up your dish and remember to use as many fruits and veggies as possible, all of the dishes that you can make with the help of this cookbook will be the healthiest and most nutritious meals that you can possibly make.

About Us

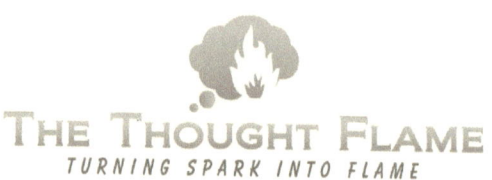

The Thought Flame is committed to add value to its customers through various books, online courses and other resources. You can learn more about us and our books at www.thethoughtflame.com.

Don't forget to check out our amazing **online video courses** at www.thethoughtflame.com/courses/ to take your knowledge to another level.

To check out our **extraordinary collection of diet/cookbooks**, visit http://www.thethoughtflame.com/category/non-fictional/cookbooks/ .

As a part of our valued relationship with our customers, we keep providing you free promotional books, courses and other stuff on subscribing with us on our site. We have a strict anti-spam policy and assure you no spam mails will be sent to your mailbox.

To subscribe with us, visit www.thethoughtflame.com.

Like our work and would like to say thanks?

Buy us a cup of coffee at www.thethoughtflame.com/coffee/

<u>Author</u>

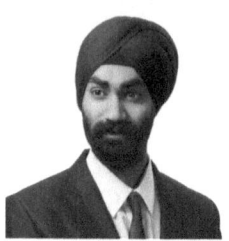

Amarpreet Singh is an avid learner and his passion for education has made him travel, work and study all across the world. He holds three masters degrees, including MBA, from top universities in Asia.

He is author of dozens of books, many of which are Amazon's bestseller, varying in various topics and categories. He also teaches many online courses having thousands of students across the world.

He has a keen interest in international affairs, economics, global poverty and politics, financial markets and entrepreneurship, and strives to be part of a community that shares the same passion.

He has worked as consultant with organizations like Airbus and The World Bank.

He loves travelling and learning about new cultures, and has been fortunate to live/work/travel/study in countries like India, China, Korea, US, South Africa, Japan, Philippines, Singapore, Canada etc., and learn about the culture and lifestyle in each of them.

To check out more of his work, visit www.thethoughtflame.com

www.ingramcontent.com/pod-product-compliance
Lightning Source LLC
Chambersburg PA
CBHW050425290526
45786CB00003B/1395